I0446567

# Qigong Exercises for Beginners

*Easy 7 Minute Qigong Routine for a Healthy Heart, Invigorate the Qi, Circulate Blood, Energies and Heal*

**Dan Phillips PhD**

# ~DEDICATION~

## ~LARRY~

For your unwavering support, encouragement, and friendship. Your presence in my life has been a constant source of inspiration. Thank you for your invaluable kindness and belief in my journey. This book is a token of appreciation for your enduring friendship and steadfast encouragement.

# TABLE OF CONTENT

CHAPTER 1. INTRODUCTION TO QIGONG AND ITS
BENEFITS:
   - EXPLAIN THE FUNDAMENTAL PRINCIPLES OF
QIGONG AND ITS HISTORICAL CONTEXT.
   - HIGHLIGHT THE BENEFITS OF PRACTICING
QIGONG, INCLUDING STRESS REDUCTION,
IMPROVED CIRCULATION, AND ENHANCED
OVERALL WELL-BEING.


CHAPTER 2. UNDERSTANDING QI AND ITS ROLE
IN HEALTH:
   - DEFINE QI AND ITS SIGNIFICANCE IN
TRADITIONAL CHINESE MEDICINE.
   - DISCUSS HOW THE CONCEPT OF QI RELATES TO
ENERGY FLOW IN THE BODY AND OVERALL
HEALTH.

## Chapter 3. Getting Started with Qigong: Preparing for Practice:

- Provide guidance on creating a suitable practice space and the importance of a calm environment.

- Explain the appropriate clothing and mindset for Qigong practice.

## Chapter 4. The 7-Minute Heart-Healthy Qigong Routine: Step-by-Step:

- Break down the 7-minute routine into individual exercises.

- Describe each exercise in detail, including posture, breathing techniques, and visualization.

## Chapter 5. Benefits of the Heart-Healthy Qigong Routine:

- Explore the specific benefits of each exercise in the routine, focusing on heart health, blood circulation, and energy flow.

- PROVIDE SCIENTIFIC EVIDENCE AND ANECDOTES THAT SUPPORT THE POSITIVE EFFECTS OF THE ROUTINE.

## CHAPTER 6. ADAPTING QIGONG FOR HEALING AND ENERGIZING:

- DISCUSS HOW THE 7-MINUTE ROUTINE CAN BE TAILORED FOR DIFFERENT PURPOSES, SUCH AS HEALING SPECIFIC AILMENTS OR INCREASING ENERGY LEVELS.
- OFFER MODIFICATIONS FOR INDIVIDUALS WITH VARYING FITNESS LEVELS OR HEALTH CONDITIONS.

## CHAPTER 7. INCORPORATING QIGONG INTO DAILY LIFE:

- PROVIDE STRATEGIES FOR INTEGRATING QIGONG PRACTICE INTO A DAILY ROUTINE, EMPHASIZING CONSISTENCY AND COMMITMENT.
- SUGGEST WAYS TO COMBINE QIGONG WITH OTHER HEALTHY HABITS FOR MAXIMUM BENEFITS.

## CHAPTER 8. ADVANCED QIGONG PRACTICES AND BEYOND:

- Introduce readers to more advanced Qigong exercises and routines for those looking to deepen their practice.

- Explore additional resources, workshops, and communities for further learning and growth in the realm of Qigong.

# CHAPTER 1

## Introduction to Qigong and its Benefits

The ancient Chinese practice of Qigong, which is based on the ideas of harmony and balance, has endured through the ages to become a widely accepted and transforming wellness method. Fundamentally, Qigong consists of a combination of deliberate breathing, soft motions, and focused purpose that work together to balance and develop Qi, the body's life force. This chapter lays the groundwork by exploring the core ideas of Qigong, outlining its historical origins, and highlighting the various advantages that practitioners of this age-old practice can obtain.

## Understanding the Foundational Ideas of Qigong:

A deep awareness of the connections between the human body, mind, and universe is fundamental to Qigong. Two core ideas of Qigong are Qi and Yin-Yang, which have their roots in traditional Chinese medicine (TCM) and ancient Chinese philosophy. Qi, sometimes referred to as life force or vital energy, nourishes every cell and organ in the body as it travels along invisible channels known as meridians. In contrast, Yin-Yang represents the duality and balance seen in nature and serves as an example of how harmony within oneself is necessary for achieving optimal well-being.

## Tracing Qigong's Historical Context:

Around 4,000 years ago, when ancient Chinese sages were looking for ways to maximize health and longevity via the harmonious alignment of body, mind, and spirit, Qigong was born. Inspired by the rhythms found in nature and by monitoring animal motions, they created workouts and meditation techniques that mirrored these organic patterns. As Qigong developed through millennia, it adapted to different schools of thought, dynasties, and geographical areas, ultimately giving rise to a variety of forms that serve a range of purposes and requirements.

**The Advantages of Qigong Practice**:
The many advantages Qigong offers its practitioners also contribute to its attraction, in addition to its historical relevance. Stress reduction is one of Qigong's most notable benefits. Encouraging practitioners to slow down, concentrate on their breathing, and do intentional movements,

Qigong offers a peaceful haven among the stresses of contemporary life. This contemplative element helps to release tension and foster inner calm, especially when combined with Qi cultivation.

Furthermore, Qigong facilitates better circulation. The fluid, soft motions encourage the body's blood and energy to move more effectively. This improved circulation provides oxygen and other essential nutrients to cells, enhancing their general vitality and supporting better organ function. The careful balancing act between breath and movement arouses and revitalizes the body's internal systems, increasing resilience.

The beneficial effects of Qigong practice extend beyond the physical body to include the mental and emotional domains. Frequent practice of Qigong cultivates mindfulness and enables practitioners to ground themselves in the present. This attentive awareness promotes a change away from regrets from the past and fears about the future, which can be a potent antidote to worry. Through cultivating this awareness, Qigong practitioners frequently report feeling better emotionally balanced and experiencing an overall sense of well-being.

Qigong has been linked to numerous health benefits in addition to stress relief and mental clarity. According to clinical research, practicing Qigong on a daily basis can assist improve cardiovascular health, lower blood pressure, and improve lung function. Its mild, low-impact characteristics also make it suitable for people of different ages and fitness levels. Regardless of age or experience level, Qigong may be customized to meet personal requirements, making it a flexible practice with a broad range of applications.

**Conclusion**

The Qigong introduction chapter prepares you for a voyage into the core of this age-old discipline. Grounded on a deep knowledge of Yin-Yang and Qi, and enhanced by millennia of experience, Qigong presents itself as an all-encompassing method of promoting health. Its numerous health benefits—ranging from better circulation and stress reduction to increased mental clarity and general well-being—attest to its continuing applicability in our fast-paced society. We are encouraged to draw on the knowledge of the past as we begin this investigation of Qigong in order to create a more wholesome and peaceful present.

# CHAPTER 2

## Understanding Qi and its Role in Health

Qi (pronounced "chee") is a key concept in traditional Chinese medicine (TCM), an age-old, all-encompassing approach to health and wellness. This chapter explores TCM's fundamental relevance of Qi and its complex understanding. We examine the theory that this essential life force circulates throughout the body, impacting general health and wellbeing.

## Characterizing Qi: The Life Force

The idea of Qi, an illusive and complex term that is difficult to translate, is central to traditional Chinese medicine. The basic life force or energy that animates all living things is frequently referred to as qi. It acts as a dynamic link between the material, psychological, and spiritual facets of life. Qi is a concept that is difficult to define or measure in terms of Western science, yet it has a significant impact on TCM theory and practice.

According to TCM, Qi is not a single thing, but rather a range of expressions that all work together to support the body and mind in harmony. Among these expressions are:

1. Yuan Qi: This is the innate Qi that each person possesses from birth; it symbolizes their health and vigor. It is comparable to the idea found in Western biology of genetic inheritance.

2. Gu Qi: Also referred to as "food Qi," Gu Qi is made up of the nutrients that are assimilated and digested. It is essential for meeting the body's daily energy requirements.

3. Zong Qi: Zong Qi is the Qi that is taken from the air by breathing, with an emphasis on the function of the lungs in dispersing this essential energy.

4. Ying Qi: In charge of providing nourishment to the organs and tissues, Ying Qi also promotes growth and healing and eases the normal operation of body systems.

5. Wei Qi: Also known as the "defensive Qi," Wei Qi strengthens the immune system's capacity to ward off disease by protecting the body from outside invaders.

## Energy Movement and Well-Being: The Role of Qi

Energy that flows freely and in balance is central to the idea of Qi. According to Traditional Chinese Medicine (TCM), good health results from Qi flowing and balancing via the body's complex system of meridians, or energy pathways. A complex system of meridians connects different tissues, organs, and physiological processes.

If Qi is flowing freely and in sufficient amounts, the body is in a balanced state that encourages life and toughness. On the other hand, imbalances caused by disruptions in Qi flow are believed to cause medical illnesses, emotional disorders, or a mix of both.

Qi equilibrium is also maintained by the interaction of two opposing but complimentary energies, Yin and Yang. Yang symbolizes the energetic, stimulating, and warming aspects, whereas Yin represents the receptive, nurturing, and cooling aspects. A person's general well-being and the uninterrupted flow of Qi depend on the harmonious balance of Yin and Yang.

**Qi and the Systems of the Body**

Comprehending Qi in relation to the body's systems offers valuable understanding of its function in preserving well-being. Let's examine the connections between Qi and a few of these systems:

Digestive System: The body uses Gu Qi, the byproduct of digestion, to meet its energy requirements. For the body to function at its best, nutrients and Qi must be properly extracted from food, which is ensured by a harmonious digestion process.

Respiratory System: Zong Qi is nourished by the air we breathe and is responsible for supporting several body systems. Zong Qi's effective circulation promotes lung health and a clear channel of energy flow throughout the body.

Circulatory System: The nourishment of the organs and tissues is mostly dependent on Ying Qi. A clear channel of Ying Qi promotes good blood flow, which makes sure that every region of the body gets the nutrition it needs.

Immune System: The free flow of Qi is essential for the body's defense against external diseases, known as Wei Qi. An immune system that is strong and has free flow of Qi is better able to prevent sickness.

Nervous System: Qi moves through a complex network of meridians that affects how the nervous system functions. Mental clarity, stress reduction, and emotional well-being are all facilitated by a regulated flow of Qi.

## Qi Disruptions and Unbalanced Health

According to TCM theory, Qi flow disturbances are frequently the cause of health imbalances. Numerous things, including as unhealthy eating habits, emotional stress, bad lifestyle decisions, and environmental influences, might cause these disruptions. There are several health problems that can arise from Qi becoming excessive, deficient, or sluggish in particular places.

1. Stagnation: A barrier or slowing down of energy flow is referred to as stagnant Qi. In the affected areas, this

may cause pain, tension, and discomfort. Mood problems and cognitive disruptions can also result from emotional and mental stagnation.

2. Deficiency: When there is not enough Qi to sustain the body's operations, there is a Qi deficiency. This may result in exhaustion, weakness, and weakened immunity, which increases the body's susceptibility to disease.

3. Excess: Conversely, an overactive or hyperactive state can result from excessive Qi. This could show up as

hyperactivity, restlessness, or anxiety symptoms.

The goal of TCM therapy for these abnormalities is to restore the normal flow of Qi. Acupuncture, herbal therapy, Qi Gong, and dietary changes are among the methods frequently used to restore Qi and enhance general health.

## Qi and Contemporary Knowledge

Despite being a fundamental component of traditional Chinese medicine for generations, the idea of Qi may appear ethereal or mystical to Western scientific minds. But more recently, studies have looked into how TCM concepts relate to contemporary knowledge, especially in the areas of energy, neurology, and mind-body relationships.

The concept of Qi is consistent with new ideas like bioelectricity, which describes the electrical signals produced by the body's tissues and cells. Additionally, psychoneuroimmunology—a study that studies the complex relationships between emotions, the neurological system, and the immunological response—and TCM's emphasis on the mind-body connection have similarities.

## Final Thoughts

A distinct viewpoint on wellbeing is provided by the comprehensive knowledge of Qi and its function in health, which bridges the gap between the mental, emotional, and spiritual facets of human existence. The way that Qi is interpreted in traditional Chinese medicine may go against established scientific paradigms in the West, but its significant impact on health and wellbeing cannot be discounted.

The idea of Qi reminds us that everything in life is interrelated, and it encourages us to take into account not just the outward signs of disease but also the underlying energetic imbalances that affect our overall health. Accepting the wisdom of Qi allows us to see health from a holistic perspective that takes into account emotions, energy, and our innate capacity for vitality.

# CHAPTER 3

**Getting Started with Qigong:**

**Preparing for Practice:**

- Provide guidance on creating a suitable practice space and the importance of a calm environment.

- Explain the appropriate clothing and mindset for Qigong practice.

Setting the stage for a successful and rewarding Qigong practice experience is essential before you begin. We'll explore the key components of a good Qigong practice in this chapter, beginning with setting up a favorable environment and developing the appropriate mindset.

## Building an Appropriate Practice Area:

Choosing a suitable practice area is essential to your Qigong practice. Locate a peaceful, clutter-free space where you may practice without interruptions. Ideally, there should be enough natural light and good ventilation in this area. An element of nature, such a view of the sky or plants, can uplift the room's general spirit. Make sure it's comfortable for you because too hot or too chilly can interfere with your concentration and Qi flow.

Even while you don't have to commit a whole room to your practice, setting up a certain area, such as a corner, can help instill a feeling of holiness and regularity in your habit. When arranging your practice area, think about adding meaningful items to add to the atmosphere, like pictures of the natural world or symbols of equilibrium.

**The Significance of a Relaxed Setting:**

A peaceful and quiet space is necessary for a successful Qigong practice. A calm, clutter-free area reduces outside distractions and promotes relaxation. Switch off or muffle electronic gadgets to prevent disruptions. If you live in a noisy neighborhood, you might want to use white noise or gentle music to provide a calming background noise.

Candlelight or low illumination are two other ways to enhance the peaceful ambiance. Recall that your practice place is a reflection of your intention to practice mindfulness and healing, not merely a physical location.

**The Right Clothes for Doing Qigong:**

When it comes to comfort and unhindered movement during your Qigong practice, clothes selection is quite important. Choose clothing that fits loosely and breathes well so that your body can move freely. Natural materials, such as cotton or bamboo, are the best since they let your skin breathe and keep you from feeling uncomfortable from being too hot.

Since most Qigong activities are done standing or with slow, gentle movements, shoes are usually not needed. You can improve your grounding experience and establish a more direct connection with the energy of the soil by practicing barefoot.

**Developing the Appropriate Mentality:**

Just as crucial as organizing your physical area is preparing your mentality. You should approach your Qigong practice with inquiry and openness. Give up any preconceived ideas and make time for yourself to be in the present. Give yourself permission to put your practice as your only priority and let go of the demands of your everyday life.

Spend a few minutes establishing your practice's intention before you start. You may do this to lower stress, enhance your well-being, or just to establish a stronger inner connection. Bring your attention to your breathing, your movements, and the sensations in your body as you progress through the exercises. Redirect your focus back to the practice if you find your thoughts straying.

**Conclusion**

The goal of preparing for a Qigong practice is to balance the mental and physical aspects in a harmonious way. Proper attire, a relaxed atmosphere, a good practice area, and the correct mindset all help to create a positive and productive experience. You can embark on a journey that not only improves your physical health but also reawakens your mind and soul in harmony with the principles of Qigong by taking care of the space where you practice. As you proceed along this path, keep in mind that the act of preparing itself can open doors to deeper transformation and connection.

# CHAPTER 4

The 7-Minute Heart-Healthy Qigong Routine: Step-by-Step:

- Break down the 7-minute routine into individual exercises.

- Describe each exercise in detail, including posture, breathing techniques, and visualization.

Gentle movements, deliberate breathing, and focused intention are all combined in the ancient Chinese practice of Qigong, which is an excellent approach to support heart health and general well-being. This is a 7-minute heart-healthy Qigong exercise that can improve energy flow, strengthen the heart, and lower stress levels. Let us examine each practice in more detail:

**Warm-up 1: Corrective Posture Situation:**

Place your feet shoulder-width apart as you stand.

2. Let your shoulders drop and flex your knees a little.

3. Lay your hands over your chest, with the palms facing up.

**Inhaling:**

Breathe deeply through your nose, feeling your chest rise and your abdomen expand. Gently release the breath through your lips, letting your chest descend.

**posture:**

With every breath, visualize a gentle, warm light coming from your heart core and permeating every part of your body.

**Exercise 2: Collecting Energy from the Sky and the Earth**

**Situation:**

1. Continue to adopt a heart-centered posture.

2. Extend your arms upwards and to the sides with your palms facing up with each inhale.

3. Bring your arms back to your chest on each exhale.

**Inhaling:**

Lift your arms and take a deep breath to absorb reviving energy from the sky. As you bring your arms down, release the air and make a connection with the energy of the earth.

**posture:**

Think of your body as a conduit connecting the nourishing solidity of the soil with the vastness of the sky. Perceive the energy circulating through you.

## Task 3: A Gently Surging Wind Dragging the Willows

### Situation:

1. Reach your arms forward to your chest from the Heart Centering Stance.

2. Maintain a flexible wrist range that permits your hands to sway slightly back and forth.

**Inhaling:**

Breathe in as your hands spread out, and out as they reunite.

**posture:**

Think of your hands and arms as dancing willow branches in the wind. Breathe with grace and fluidity when you move.

**Practice 4: Knock Softly on the Door of Life**

**Situation:**

Bring your arms down to your sides.

2. Using your hands, form loose fists.

**Inhaling:**

Breathe in while bringing your fists up to your chest and maintaining a relaxed elbow position. Breathe out and tap your chest lightly, concentrating on your sternum.

**posture:**

Envision yourself knocking on your body's door of energy and wellbeing. Your chest should resonate with the mild vibrations.

**Embracing the Tree of Life is the fifth exercise.**

## Situation:

1. Spread your arms wide and turn your palms outward.
2. Bend your knees slightly and visualize giving a tree trunk a hug.

## Inhaling:

Spread your arms and take a breath, bringing in new life. Breathe out as you re-enter and release any trapped energy.

## posture:

Imagine yourself deeply embedded in the ground, drawing nourishment from the earth like a tree. Feel the inner solidity and power of the tree.

## Exercise 6: Stretch Your Heart

### Situation:

1. With your palms facing each other, extend your arms forward to chest level.

2. Take a deep breath in and extend your arms to the sides, gently stretching your chest.

### Inhaling:

Breathe in while you spread your arms wide and widen your heart center. As you reunite your arms, let a breath.

**posture:**

With every breath, visualize your heart center opening up and allowing love, joy, and vitality to freely flow through it.

Workout 7: Seizing and Sealing Qi

Situation:

1. With your palms facing down, bring your arms down to your sides.

2. Maintain a solid footing position.

Inhaling:

Take a deep breath and see energy building in your lower dantian, which is the energy center directly beneath your navel. Sealing the energy inside, exhale as you bring your hands to your lower dantian.

**posture:**

Imagine that the breath and movements from the preceding exercises have refreshed a radiant ball of energy at your lower dantian. Experience balance and harmony within.

**Final Thoughts**

This 7-minute heart-healthy Qigong exercise provides a potent, yet straightforward, method to improve your cardiovascular health and develop a closer relationship with your body's energy. By integrating deliberate breathing, conscious movement, and visualization, you may stimulate your heart center, ease tension, and encourage the free flow of Qi. Add this practice to your daily routine to reap the heart-healthy and general well-being advantages of Qigong.

# CHAPTER 5

**Benefits of the Heart-Healthy**

**Qigong Routine:**

- Explore the specific benefits of each exercise in the routine, focusing on heart health, blood circulation, and energy flow.

- Provide scientific evidence and anecdotes that support the positive effects of the routine.

For those seeking the highest level of health and energy, the Heart-Healthy Qigong Routine is a guiding light. This chapter explores the many advantages that each activity in the regimen provides, focusing on the effects on heart health, blood circulation, and energy flow. As we learn more about the complex interactions between body, mind, and spirit, the transforming impacts of this routine—backed by both scientific data and anecdotal evidence—become evident.

First Workout: Promoting Heart Health:

The Heart's gently opening exerciseHealthy Qigong Practice establishes the foundation for heart health. This workout promotes optimal function by stimulating blood flow and gently massaging the heart through its rhythmic motions and focused breathing. Regular Qigong practice has been linked to lowered blood pressure and a lower risk of heart disease, according to scientific studies. The integration of movement with intentional focus cultivates a balanced symbiosis between the cardiac energy and physical components, advancing overall health.

workout 2: Increasing Blood Flow:

The emphasis moves to the critical function of blood circulation as we go on to the second exercise. This exercise's flowing motions promote blood's easy passage through the vessels, improving the body's ability to supply nutrients and oxygen to every cell. Enhanced circulation promotes overall energy and organ health. Anecdotal accounts of consistent practice of this exercise frequently mention feeling more energised and with greater warmth in the extremities.

Workout 3: Stimulating Qi Movement:

The third exercise, which focuses on energizing the body's Qi flow, is the core of the regimen. This exercise improves the flow of life energy along the meridians by combining movement, breath, and intention in a dynamic way. This promotes a balanced and harmonious state of being. Stories abound about how regular practice leads to more energy, greater mental clarity, and a deep sense of vitality.

Workout 4: Enriching the Mind-Body Bond:

The routine's fourth exercise strengthens the link between heart health and mental wellness. Stress reduction and emotional equilibrium are promoted by this activity, which leads practitioners to connect with their heart center. Research has shown that Qigong has a beneficial effect on the autonomic nervous system, which lowers stress hormone levels and elevates mood. Anecdotal data suggests that consistent participation in this practice leads to an increased sense of inner peace and emotional resilience.

Workout 5: Reestablishing Energetic Balance:

Between the previous motions and the end of the practice, the penultimate exercise acts as a transition. Its main goal is to bring about an energetic balance again, letting any trapped Qi release and flow freely. Feelings of lightness and equilibrium are typically experienced after this exercise, which supports the idea that Qigong not only supports physical health but also nourishes the spirit.

**Sealing and Integrating:**

The Heart-Healthy Qigong Routine's last exercise integrates all of its advantages and restores a sense of wholeness, sealing the practice. Body, mind, and spirit can be harmonized with this technique that draws the hands to the Dantian, the body's energy center. Practitioners who complete this closing exercise frequently describe feeling deeply connected and grounded.

**Conclusion**

The Heart-Healthy Qigong Routine demonstrates the complex relationship that exists between energy flow, physical movement, and overall health. Every exercise promotes heart health, better blood flow, and increased energy flow, all of which lead to a more complete feeling of vigor. Underpinned by empirical evidence and firsthand accounts, this regimen's transformational potential extends beyond the physical domain to encompass emotional equilibrium and spiritual congruence. Embrace the deep rewards that await you as you set out on your adventure to synchronize the rhythm of your heart with the universe.

# CHAPTER 6

Adapting Qigong for Healing and Energizing:
- Discuss how the 7-minute routine can be tailored for different purposes, such as healing specific ailments or increasing energy levels.
- Offer modifications for individuals with varying fitness levels or health conditions.

Qigong is a flexible practice that can be tailored to meet individual health goals and energy requirements because of its gentle movements, concentrated breathing, and awareness. The seven-minute Qigong exercise can be tailored to target various conditions, such as boosting vitality or curing particular illnesses. Changes can also be made to accommodate those with different degrees of fitness or medical issues.

**Treating Particular Illnesses:**

Cardiovascular Health: To concentrate on circulation and heart health, give special attention to movements that gently open and extend the chest, including Flowing Breeze Sways the Willows and the Heart-Opening Stretch. Imagine that with every action, your heart gets stronger and more resilient. Breathing slowly and deeply can improve blood flow and relaxation, which benefits the cardiovascular system.

tension and Anxiety: Pay close attention to exercises like the Heart Centering Stance and Gathering Earth and Sky Energy that include deep, conscious breathing and relaxation in order to manage tension and anxiety. Include deeper exhalations to trigger the body's relaxation response and see stress dissipating with each breath.

Digestive Issues: To aid with digestion, concentrate on abdominal exercises that feature soft twists or movements, like Gathering and Sealing Qi and Flowing Breeze Sways the Willows. As you move, visualize your digestive system operating easily and effectively. Use abdominal breathing to stimulate and massage your digestive system.

**Raising Vitality Levels:**

Fatigue and Low Energy: Add more vigorous and dynamic movements to your routine to increase your energy levels. Increase the speed of several exercises, such as Heart-Opening Stretch and Flowing Breeze Sways the Willows, to activate the body's energy and vitality. Imagine yourself taking in and assimilating bright energy from the universe.

Morning Wake-Up Routine: As a reviving morning habit, follow the 7-minute routine. Stretch gently at first, and throw open your arms to greet the new day. To awaken the body and mind, change the practice to incorporate more dynamic movements and rapid breathing, such as lightly bouncing on your toes during the Heart-Opening Stretch.

## Adjustments for Various Health Conditions and Fitness Levels:

Novices and Elderly: Proceed with the exercise more slowly if you are a beginner or have limited movement. Limit your range of motion when performing exercises like the Willows' Flowing Breeze and Heart-Opening Stretch. Make sure to keep your breathing deep and under control and your posture correct. If necessary, use a strong chair for support.

Physical Restrictions: Those who are limited by their physical condition might modify the regimen by completing the exercises while seated. For instance, when seated, perform the Heart-Opening Stretch by gently stretching your arms out in front of you. Breathwork and visualization are still essential tools for healing and energy channeling.

Chronic Health Conditions: Before starting a new fitness program, those with chronic health conditions should speak with their healthcare practitioners. Modify the regimen in accordance with personal capacities and medical advice. Exercises that encourage attention, calm, and moderate movement should be your main focus.

## Final Thoughts

The flexibility and accessibility of Qigong are what make it so beautiful. Through customization of the 7-minute routine to individual healing objectives or energy requirements, as well as adjustments for differing levels of fitness and medical conditions, practitioners can reap the significant advantages of this approach. Qigong becomes an individualized tool to cultivate energy, enhance well-being, and support healing, all while respecting the individuality of each person's path toward balance and health. As with any new fitness regimen, it's crucial to pay attention to your body, practice carefully, and, if needed, seek advice from trained instructors or medical specialists.

# CHAPTER 7

**Incorporating Qigong into Daily Life:**

- Provide strategies for integrating Qigong practice into a daily routine, emphasizing consistency and commitment.

- Suggest ways to combine Qigong with other healthy habits for maximum benefits.

Qigong's transforming power is shown at its core, but integrating this age-old practice into contemporary life is a struggle. This chapter explores the practice of integrating Qigong into daily life and provides techniques to guarantee dedication, regularity, and a peaceful coexistence of Qigong with other health-promoting practices. The path to improved well-being develops into a way of life rather than merely a routine.

**First Strategy: Begin Small, Develop Consistency:**

Since time can be a valuable resource, start by allocating a tiny amount of your day to Qigong. A few minutes every morning or evening can make a big difference. Maintaining consistency is essential because the cumulative benefits of consistent practice outweigh the benefits of infrequent, intense sessions. Choose a reasonable objective that works with your schedule, and as your commitment becomes more firm, progressively increase it.

## Method 2: Establish Customs and Practices:

To improve Qigong's incorporation into your routine, incorporate it into your already-existing daily rituals. Associating Qigong with normal tasks strengthens its significance, whether you're incorporating it into your morning routine or using it as a way to wind down before bed. A feeling of familiarity and expectation can be fostered by designating a certain time and location for practice.

**Modern Approach 3: Adopting Mindful Multitasking:**

There are times when mindful multitasking can be helpful, even though mindfulness requires complete focus on the practice. Easy Qigong poses can be done on your daily commute, while you're waiting in line, or even during brief breaks. These mini-sessions help you fit in little moments of relaxation and renewal throughout your day without interfering with your plans.

**Combining Qigong with Other Healthful Habits: Strategy 4:**

Make a peaceful union with other practices that improve health, such as Qigong. When Qigong is combined with other disciplines like yoga, meditation, or even a healthy diet, the effects of both are enhanced. The synergy produced by these complimentary movements supports Qigong's all-encompassing approach to wellbeing.

## Strategy 5: Create a Community and Accountability System

Establishing a practice group or enrolling in a Qigong class can promote community and accountability. Your dedication to regular practice can be strengthened by sharing experiences, receiving updates on your progress, and having the chance to discuss ideas with other practitioners. The support and friendship of a community may keep you committed even in the face of adversity.

## Method 6: Foster Mindful Awareness Outside of Practice:

Apply the mindfulness that is developed via Qigong practice to other facets of your everyday life. It is possible to apply the awareness of breath, body sensations, and intention to everyday tasks like eating, walking, and social interaction with ease. The advantages of Qigong are enhanced by this extension of attention, resulting in a more harmonious and comprehensive way of living.

**Rendering:**

Adding Qigong to your everyday routine is an activity that goes beyond routine transformation. By incorporating Qigong with other health-promoting techniques, integrating it strategically, and practicing mindful multitasking, you may transform this age-old art form into a dynamic part of your overall well-being. You can develop both physical health and a stronger sense of self and community by adopting these techniques and incorporating them into your daily life. Once you integrate Qigong into your everyday routine, you start a path towards ongoing energy and harmony.

# CHAPTER 8

**Advanced Qigong Practices and Beyond:**

- Introduce readers to more advanced Qigong exercises and routines for those looking to deepen their practice.

- Explore additional resources, workshops, and communities for further learning and growth in the realm of Qigong.

Advanced exercises and resources are available for those who want to deepen their practice and learn more about Qigong, taking their journey to new heights. As you continue on your Qigong path, you'll discover that this age-old discipline offers an extensive array of methods, ideas, and encounters that can improve your mental, emotional, and spiritual health. In this section, we walk you through advanced Qigong exercises and provide you to more resources for your further education and development.

## Advanced Practices and Exercises for Qigong:

1. Wu Qin Xi's Five Animal Frolics:
The Five Animal Frolics are a kind of martial arts and ancient Chinese medicine that mimic the movements and habits of particular animals, including tigers, deer, bears, monkeys, and cranes. The motions of each animal align with particular organs and meridians, fostering flexibility, balance, and energy flow.

2. Zhan Zhuang's Standing Pole Qigong:
This is a static kind of Qigong where you hold different positions for long

periods of time. It develops rootedness, balance, and inner strength. You can cultivate a profound sense of energy circulation and attention with Standing Pole Qigong.

3. Seven Corsets (Ba Duan Jin):
This eight-exercise series targets particular body parts to improve general health. It includes breathing exercises, visualization, and dynamic stretching to support both physical and mental well-being.

4. Orbit Meditation in Microcosms:
The goal of this sophisticated technique is to move energy via the "microcosmic orbit," which is a

channel connecting the spine's energy centers. It raises the practitioner's level of spiritual and energetic awareness while assisting in the Yin and Yang energy balance.

**Resources for Additional Education and Development:**

**1. Retreats and Workshops in Qigong:**

Immersion learning opportunities can be obtained by participating in seminars and retreats facilitated by seasoned Qigong teachers. These gatherings provide chances for guided practices, in-depth instruction, and networking with other like-minded practitioners.

## 2. Stories and Online Materials:

Comprehensive instructions and insights into advanced Qigong practices can be found in a plethora of books, websites, and online courses. Examine the creations of well-known Qigong masters like Yang Jwing-Ming, Ken Cohen, and Mantak Chia.

## 3. Approved Teachers:

Look for qualified Qigong instructors online or in your community. Whether you take classes in person or virtually, you can get individualized advice and correction to make sure you're using advanced techniques correctly.

## 4. Schools of Traditional Chinese Medicine (TCM):

Comprehensive training programs that explore Qigong practices, energy healing, and the theories that drive them are offered by numerous TCM institutions and holistic health facilities.

5. Retreats focusing on mindfulness and meditation:

By promoting inner awareness, mental clarity, and a stronger connection with your body's energy, taking part in mindfulness and meditation retreats can enhance your Qigong practice.

6. Online Forums and Communities:

Make connections with other Qigong practitioners by joining social media groups and online forums. Talking with others, exchanging stories, and asking for guidance can all yield insightful and helpful information.

**Fostering a Lifelong Path:**

Recall that your path is an ongoing process as you delve into more complex Qigong techniques and access higher levels of consciousness. A lifetime journey of self-discovery, healing, and transformation is provided by qigong. Honor the wisdom of your body, be receptive to new experiences, and welcome the profound connections that Qigong can reveal between mind, body, and spirit. You'll continue to discover the benefits of this age-old practice via commitment, perseverance, and a voracious appetite for knowledge, which will enhance your life and wellbeing in ways you would never have dreamed of.

www.ingramcontent.com/pod-product-compliance
Lightning Source LLC
Chambersburg PA
CBHW072336290526
45794CB00002B/901